HUNGRY FOR WELLNESS

Elsie Taylor

This book is dedicated to the patients, friends, and family
who sought options to improve their health status
and asked me for advice regarding most of the common health
issues.

If not for them, this book probably would not exist.

CONTENTS

INTRODUCTION

HUNGRY FOR WELLNESS
Integrating a new Medical paradigm

My first teacher was my mother, Elvie Taylor. She influenced, and continues to influence, how I practice medicine—and, most importantly, how I interact with individuals.

My mom devoted much of her life supporting community efforts to improve all aspects of the human condition. She was a devout Christian, who brought her evangelism into the California prison system in Susanville, California, near the town of Herlong, where I was born. My mom grew up on a plantation in the rural south, in Arkansas and Louisiana, and nature's remedies were well known to her. She, along with my father, applied herbal principles to treat their children's various colds and childhood illnesses. This practical approach was effective in nearly every situation; and to this day, my siblings and I do not suffer from high blood pressure, diabetes, or heart disease.

A total optimist, my mother exuded a positive presence in every social setting. I once had a fiancé who spoke of her in the most admirable way. "In this 'Peyton Place' environment," he said, "your mom is the only person in town that no one speaks of in a negative manner. Everyone speaks of her with much respect and admiration." She died much too young, at the age of 40.

My mom has continued to influence my interaction with others, especially as a healthcare professional. In the beginning of my work with patients, while residing in Oakland, California as a single parent of a then-four-year-old son, and being a full-time student in nursing school, I worked a couple of hours weekly on the healthcare van, which provided free healthcare to the homeless. I did this outside of the nursing training, moved by the desire to provide care whenever and wherever I could make a contribution.

I read recently how a woman is offering a class in knitting to prison inmates. In terms of healing, what is interesting to me is that this class is considered the most popular course offered at that particular prison. The inmates have to maintain their best behavior as a prerequisite to attend the class. This speaks volumes to the fact that if you treat people with respect in a non-judgmental manner, you establish an environment where they flourish.

I had already been exposed to this view from the effects of my mom's prison-ministry. It was clear to me that the spiritual component is not separate from the body-healing component, in caring for persons needing healing. As a health professional in adulthood, I thought that it should be possible to link the importance of looking at the whole person with the dynamics that lead to chronic illness, mental illness, and stress—the "mind-body-soul" connection. Ongoing stress, for example, increases the release of cortisol, one of the stress hormones, which can elevate blood sugar, increase blood pressure, and even induce insomnia. I was certain that reducing people's inner torment could contribute to their healing. I was not surprised at my mom's successes in her prison ministry. Even her soft voice was therapeutic.

My approach to the delivery of medical care is holistic. The traditional Western medical-care model is limited in providing care that addresses the need to support the whole person. I acquired a first-hand appreciation for a more comprehensive holistic approach while working in medical practices that support this kind of model. My first job as a Registered Nurse was in Oncology in a hospital in San Francisco, California, working primarily with bone-marrow-transplant patents. An innovative medical-delivery model called "Plane Tree" was incorporated into this hospital unit. This concept was developed by a patient who had a very bad experience while in a hospital following the model of traditional allopathic medicine. In contrast, the Plane Tree model included:

- soothing classical music,
- fresh-cut floral bouquets, replenished weekly,
- original art work,
- wood furniture in the patients' rooms and about the unit,
- a library with educational DVDs and books,
- a personal chef in a fully equipped kitchen,
- and a massage therapist to treat patients and staff members.

Many cancer patients had to experience extended hospital stays, and having a more home-like environment promoted a less stressful stay.

While attending Stanford University's Primary Care Physician Assistant program in the early 1990s, I acquired a broader medical education that included Complementary and Integrated theories. (A Physician Assistant can work independently of a physician, as long as there is an avenue to communicate promptly in case of an emergency situation. We are trained by physicians to perform 90 percent of their work.) The Complementary/Integrative medical model is a blend of traditional medical practices that also includes practices not considered components of Western medical healthcare delivery—for example, energy medicine, healing touch, and herbal remedies, as well as procedures now considered mainstream, such as acupuncture. One of the program directors was studying Alternative Medicine for her Ph.D., and she shared principles of Integrative Medicine with those of us in the program who were interested.

Later, I was offered the opportunity to work as a Physician's Assistant in Minnesota, as a primary care provider in two start-up Public Housing Clinics. Ninety percent of the patients at one site were Hmong residents from Cambodia and Laos. This was a great opportunity for me to learn endogenous (or native folk medicine) practices, which usually include herbal remedies, while coordinating with a tribal Shaman.

What I found was that the more enlightened patients were willing to try healing modes outside the usual Western model and to apply theories of herbal supplements, foods that heal, and energy medicine to aid them in improving body functions. Indeed, many people who have tried to manage a chronic illness using traditional Western medical applications are finding that their condition does not improve. In some cases, it even worsens, due to the limits of just ingesting chemicals to manage their disease. For these and similar reasons, an increasing number of people have begun to seek out more effective tactics to help them manage their illness when traditional Western medical practices fall short of their expectations.

The advantage of Integrative medicine is that it incorporates modalities that promote healing via nutritional support, herbal remedies, energy medicine, spiritual support, and many other alternative techniques.

Part I

Weight Loss

"PLEASE HELP ME LOSE WEIGHT"

This is a very common request of so many patients of all ages.

Because the loss of a few extra pounds around the midriff is the common denominator that leads to the reduction of many other health problems, after getting frequent requests from my patients for help in losing weight, I began to compile a list of many of the remedies that helped to reduce back pain and to lower elevated blood pressure or high blood-sugar levels. I would write down recommendations for a variety of health problems on Post-it-Notes. Weeks later, the patient would return with better-than-expected results. (In fact, this is one of the motivating factors that led me to write this book.)

I'll briefly share with you a situation that prompted me to impart as much information to as many people as possible in a very short time.

About six months ago, I had an opportunity to ride the Greyhound bus from Los Angeles to Santa Cruz, California. I chose to catch a late-night bus so that I would arrive back in Santa Cruz before 10 AM the following morning, in time for work. For the first two hours I thought the trip would be easy and totally non-eventful. But as midnight approached, that delusion was promptly quashed.

I was sitting in the window seat; the bus was only half-full. A young man, who appeared to weigh about 350 pounds, asked me if the aisle seat was available. I thought, "Oh well, there go my plans to enjoy at least five hours of uninterrupted sleep" as the young man took the adjoining seat. I began to drift off to sleep, when suddenly a mass seemed to engulf the left half of my body. The large person sitting next to me had fallen into a deep sleep; and as his body relaxed, it began to occupy space far into my seat zone. Since it was not my intent to make him feel bad about occupying more than his share of the bus, I gave him a soft jab in the elbow. He woke up and promptly corrected his positioning—but now he blocked part of the aisle. I began to feel that I should remain awake the duration of the trip: after all, I wasn't sure that the other passengers were certified in, or as proficient in, CPR as I was. I had to deliver a few subtle jabs each time he dozed off into a deep sleep, and I felt so bad for him. When we were about 15 minutes from the next bus terminal, I overheard him phone for a cab and I was very relieved. Although I felt I should have apologized for interrupting his naps, it would have been difficult to verbalize what was probably an awkward encounter for us both, at best.

Back at work, realizing more urgently how important it is to attain a healthy weight, I wrote down brief health-care tips on Post-It notes in response to questions patients would ask me (frequently including, "How can I lose weight?"). I then gave the Post-It Notes to the staff to translate. While this worked, it proved to be very time consuming, and not very practical in a busy clinical-practice setting. Noticing that many of the tips I gave out covered the same or a similar topic, I decided to make things easier by making photocopies of my notes (once translated), and handing them out to a variety of patients. The results were good! This showed me that patients are more compliant with health-care recommendations when they clearly understand the theory behind the recommendation.

Many of my patients' health concerns are based directly on the well-known correlation between chronic illness and obesity. Most people are aware of the statistics that show an increase in the number of people with Type 2 Diabetes and heart disease. *Prevention of obesity is the key intervention if we want to improve our health, especially the health of young people.* It is easier to avoid becoming overweight than it is to lose the extra pounds acquired.

So that you, too, can benefit, here are some of the tips that I have shared with patients, friends, and family.

1. **Exercise:** One of the most challenging obstacles to weight management is when a person has suffered some type of injury to the musculoskeletal system, making it difficult to exercise at the level necessary to avoid weight gain. Here are some excellent ways to exercise for weight control:

- **Walking:** A brisk 30-minute walk every day will keep the weight under better control.
- **Swimming:** Swimming is a great alternative workout, as it incorporates cardio- and muscle-toning. You must move to lose excess weight and maintain overall good health. A 30-minute swim will provide this.
- **Jumping rope or on a trampoline:** This increases the bone-building cycle.

2. **Sauna:** Try visiting a spa that has an *infrared sauna*. The benefit is that you lose weight while just sitting there. This type of sauna promotes the removal of heavy metals from the body. There are a number of chronic illnesses that implicate heavy-metal toxins in their development. Most heavy metals bind to fat cells. Heavy metals are stored mostly in adipose tissue (fat cells). When you raise the rate of metabolism by way of increased exercise, supplements/medications, or Infra-red sauna, you effectively mobilize fat cells and ultimately aid in weight loss as the body releases toxins. Infrared sauna treatments also reduce cholesterol, arthritic inflammation, and pain.

3. **Drink lots of water—but not with meals:** Drink a large amount of water in the morning upon awakening, even before you brush your teeth. However, do not consume beverages, including water, while eating a meal. This is because beverages dilute the digestive enzymes that are available to digest and assimilate nutrients from the foods you consume. After age 25-30, the amount of digestive enzymes available to digest our foods diminishes to 40-60 percent. In this case, digestive enzymes must be added to the diet. Properly functioning digestive enzymes play a part in keeping a healthy weight. As more nutrients are released from foods, the brain sends out signals that you can stop eating, now that adequate nutrients have been delivered into the bloodstream. Then, a few hours later, blood-sugar

levels become low and signal that you must eat to restore them to balance.

4. **Drink Bragg's vinegar and white grape juice shortly before meals:** I suggest that people mix equal amounts of Bragg's vinegar and white grape juice (about 3 tablespoons of each), and drink this mixture about 5 minutes before consuming a meal. When you consume something that's bitter, you stimulate the back of the tongue, which then activates the hydrochloric acid pump. These digestive enzymes will aid in the digestion of your meal, and the absorption of nutrients from the small intestines into the bloodstream.

5. **Avoid drinking a large amount of cow's milk.** Excess milk produces a high acid content in the stomach, which causes calcium to be extracted from the bones to neutralize the acid content.

6. **Do a colon cleanse:** A 30-day colon cleanse provides several benefits: (a) it removes excess mucus toxins that interfere with full nutrient absorption; and (b) it reduces cravings—the brain detects the presence of nutrients that are needed, and sends signals to stop eating because the body has now received the nutrients it requires to provide energy for body function. The addition of a detoxify-cleanse for the colon, liver, spleen, and kidney will improve immunity, brain function, and energy levels—and also promote weight loss.

7. **Probiotic:** Take a broad-spectrum probiotic to destroy Candida Albicans, which is yeast that proliferates when we take an antibiotic. The Candida organism is known as an "opportunistic bug," in that it grows out of control when the beneficial bacteria that are needed to metabolize foods—the normal flora (the normal composition of elements contained in our gut)—are destroyed. Candida, being a yeast organism, requires sugar in order to survive.

The overgrowth of Candida increases carbohydrate cravings, causes bloating, gas production, poor digestion, fatigue, and depression. Many females complain of a vaginal yeast infection after taking antibiotics as prescribed, due to the proliferation of the "opportunistic bug."

8. **Balance proteins with carbohydrates and healthy fats:** Always consume a protein with a carbohydrate and healthy fats in equal proportions. This is because when you eat a carbohydrate, insulin is released from the pancreas to maintain normal blood-sugar levels. The release of insulin into the bloodstream triggers the storage of fat as an energy reserve. In order to manage weight long term, and maintain optimum health, the body requires: carbohydrates, for energy; protein, to build and maintain muscle- and organ-tissue stability; vegetables, for energy in the form of enzymes; and a source of fiber, to promote elimination of toxins and other waste products.

As an illustration: I took care of a patient who came to an urgent-care center. She was concerned that she had a bladder infection, because for about the last two days, she had had to urinate every 30 minutes. The urine sample we obtained from her was normal, but the level of protein was dangerously elevated. I asked what she had been eating. She answered that she had consumed a steak and eggs, 3 times per day for the past 10 days, in an effort to lose weight. Although she had successfully lost about 7 pounds in only 10 days, she already had signs of minor kidney damage due to the excessive protein intake without the balance of carbohydrates. This is because the kidney is not designed to use animal protein as its primary energy source. So a balance of proteins with carbohydrates and healthy fats is essential.

9. **Do resistance training:** Resistance training increases muscle mass. The increase in muscle mass will increase the resting metabolism, and therefore the amount of calories burned. When my patients cry in dismay that "I only lost a couple of

pounds in a week, in spite of all my exercise and calorie restriction," I have to remind them that muscle weighs more than fat. That's why I often encourage clients to measure their waist circumference. When I then ask, "Do your pants [or skirt] fit the same as before?" they usually beam with pride, indicating that, yes, their clothes do indeed have a looser fit.

Obesity and Children

I have worked with a program in Beverly Hills designed to address the obesity epidemic in children. This program included a well-rounded approach, incorporating a medical evaluation, a weekly consultation regarding best food choices, and a personal trainer who took the children through their weekly paces. My role in this setting was to perform an initial physical exam, and to review lab tests with both the child and the parent, and to provide recommendations for a shopping list and menus that the entire family could live with. In most cases, the entire family (not only the children in question) benefitted from these adjustments, lost weight, and improved their overall health. In some instances, the adults in the family experienced a drop in their blood pressure, a reduction in their cholesterol levels, and in some cases a reversal in Type 2 diabetes. I addressed the whole family's diet because it was important that the children not feel as though they were a separate entity from the rest of the family, and it was much more practical to prepare meals that the entire family would consume.

I also provided guidance to children with eating disorders—both with those who were unable to gain weight, as well as those with extreme eating disorders, such as Prader Willi syndrome. (Prader Willi syndrome is a genetic disorder where the child exhibits severe obsessive-compulsive behavior, stubborn lack of discipline, and obesity. The situation can get so extreme that the guardian/parents of these children must place locks on the doors of the refrigerator and shelves where any foods are stored.) Of course, the incidence of people with severe eating disorders is relatively low when you compare the numbers of people who are overweight or obese.

The percentage of Americans who have been diagnosed with other eating disorders (such as bulimia or anorexia nervosa) is statistically low in relation to the percentage that suffers from obesity. The best approach for addressing the growing numbers of people with expanding waistlines is to use an evaluation tool to determine if there are any medical problems that must first be corrected. This includes physical restrictions due to injury, or congenital problems that would require mechanical support to increase caloric expenditure, as well as restrict caloric intake. The next step is to explore behavior patterns that predispose some people to be more prone to holding onto those extra pounds.

Women: "Muscle Up" to Increase Metabolism

The more muscle mass you build, the more calories you burn with less effort. And most females don't have the lean muscle mass of most males. However, not everyone has the ability to build massive muscles; and females do prefer to attain a softer contour.

In a weight management clinic, rule number one is that you don't want to upset the milieu by comparing a woman's weight-loss effort to a man's. Males have higher levels of testosterone. Neither gender will build muscle when testosterone level is in the lower-than-normal range.

In our initial consultation, I ask my female clients to perform 60 push-ups or 40 pull-ups twice weekly. If looks could kill, I would already be lifeless. However, I then go on to explain that I understand how absurd the request, might seem, but, that is the ultimate target goal they might aspire to achieve.

Recipe for Lean Muscle-Mass

Here is the one recipe that will help you develop more lean muscle-mass, no matter what your metabolic type may be. This has been effective for most of my clients, friends, and relatives who could adhere to the meal plan.

> 2 cups baby spinach
> 2 cups "Spring mix" salad greens
> 2 Tablespoons raw pecans
> 2 hard-boiled eggs
> 2 Tablespoons dried cranberries
> Bragg's vinegar, olive oil, chopped garlic*

*The vinaigrette dressing for the salad can have poultry, fish, or quinoa, or 3-4 ounces of protein for females and 7-8 ounces for males.

A Final Word of Encouragement

You must *move* to lose weight. And in order to control weight for a *lifetime,* you must increase metabolism by increasing muscle mass. If you follow the tips in this section, you will be in good shape all the way around!

WEIGHT MANAGEMENT AND HORMONES

Weight management is not only a challenge for a great number of people, but it is also the primary factor affecting the health status of millions of individuals. Most folks understand that when those extra pounds are shed, many health problems that are connected to some illnesses are reversed.

That's right. By losing weight, you also will free yourself from problems such as diabetes (with its requirement of constant blood tests), serious heart disease, and high blood pressure. Get rid of those extra pounds, and you will experience renewed energy.

I want to share some practical tips with you that I've shared with people for years as a Registered Nurse, Physician Assistant and Metabolic Typing coach. I have imparted this information to people looking to shed some pounds, as well as to reverse high blood pressure, high cholesterol, and Type 2 diabetes. The best news of all is that this is not that hard to do, once you understand what is going on in your body and do simple things to correct your weight.

But before we get into those tips, we need to look at certain *hormones*—especially their connection to stress and to being overweight.

STRESS =
Slows down metabolism
Tight, tense muscles
Rapid, pounding heartbeat
Elevated blood pressure
Slows down body's ability to repair
Stimulates weight gain

You can see that excessive negative stress is not good for the body, or for attaining and maintaining an ideal weight. Let's take a look at how certain hormones come into the picture.

Cortisol

Cortisol is a hormone released from the adrenal glands to provide us with the energy to get up and get on with our daily activities. *Excess stress causes higher cortisol levels, and inhibits weight loss.*

Cortisol peaks in the morning, between about 8AM until about 12 noon, and is at its lowest ebb from about 10 PM until 2AM—about the time that the liver begins to undergo its restorative process. In highly stressful situations, *cortisol is released at much higher levels.* That is why it's known as "the stress hormone," or "the fight or flight hormone." In order to manage this confrontation with stress, extra fuel or an energy surge is required to bring more blood and oxygen to the brain to enhance vision, and to bring extra blood, oxygen, and glucose to the legs to increase their ability to run faster than in a normal situation. This is where extra cortisol comes in handy.

However, if you don't burn up that extra fuel rapidly by running or fighting (fight or flight), then cortisol will convert from a sugar molecule into adipose (fat)—fat with a propensity to settle around the gut and the buttocks. So prolonged or frequent cortisol surges can place more fat in the places you least care to have it stored.

Other Effects of Cortisol

- Cortisol affects the heart, blood vessels, blood pressure, water excretion, and electrolyte balance. (Electrolytes are minerals, such as potassium, sodium, and magnesium)

- Cortisol mobilizes protein in body tissues, and moves fatty acids from adipose (fat)—stored in storage deposits throughout the body—deep into the abdominal area. That is why we see the enlarged abdominal girth.

- Cortisol helps cells produce antibodies to support immune function, and works to reduce inflammation.

- Cortisol affects the eyes and the gastrointestinal tract. Visual acuity will improve, but only momentarily; and the muscles of the legs also receive a surge of oxygen by way of increased blood flow. (This is a negative feedback mechanism held over from caveman days when men had to hunt their meal or run from an attacking animal.)

- It affects mood, behavior, and other central-nervous-system functions.

Modifying Our Response to Stress

We can't dodge the stressors of living, but we *can* modify our response to stress. One really important way to protect ourselves from excessive stress is to get enough sleep. *Sleep deprivation elevates both our cortisol level and our blood pressure.* Fibromyalgia patients, for example, have an inversion in their cortisol levels, which tend to peak at night and are at their lowest level in the morning. This may be one reason why many patients with Fibromyalgia are insomniacs, and suffer from chronic fatigue as well as muscle and joint aches, as the liver attempts to revitalize the body when its biorhythms are disrupted.

Perhaps the most relevant aspect of cortisol, for the purpose of this section on weight, is that *when it is released in excessive levels and/or for a prolonged duration, it will promote weight gain.*

This is why cortisol is known as the "death hormone." If levels of cortisol are released at very high levels for a long period of time, this will cause the breakdown of every tissue in the body. If your levels of cortisol are extremely lower than normal levels, your basic metabolism slows down considerably, leading to chronic health disorders. Eventually, if metabolism halts, death occurs.

How Do We Get a Handle on Cortisol?

- **Get enough sleep to reduce stress**—ideally, 6 to 8 hours of deep, uninterrupted sleep.
- **Exercise:** aerobic exercise, cardio, and resistance or weight-lifting techniques that don't require expensive exercise equipment.

- **Relaxation:** Meditation, Qi Gung, and yoga promote relaxation and increase agility. Reflexology for the hands and feet is also helpful.

DHEA (dehydroepiandrosterone): The Anti-Stress, Energy-boosting Hormone

DHEA is a "good" hormone, also released from the adrenal glands, that assists in maintaining energy and resistance to stress. It is released to help repair the tissue breakdown caused by **cortisol.** **DHEA**, along with human growth hormone and other hormones, repair and rebuild muscle and other body tissue while you are asleep. This is one reason why it's so important to get sufficient sleep.

People who are involved in "extreme sports" get a "natural high" when engaging in these activities—indeed, they deliberately induce this "good stress" precisely in order to experience this euphoric state. However, when the stress response is extended, it can lead to exhaustion. We then no longer release the cortisol levels needed to adapt, and our DHEA levels drop. Prolonged stress also can cause depletion in Vitamin C, the B vitamins, and minerals that are essential in supporting our immune system.

DHEA is a precursor to testosterone. Inadequate levels of testosterone will render it nearly impossible to attain greater lean-muscle mass. Increasing muscle mass will also increase metabolism. It is also very important to *maintain* muscle mass, since after our thirties we lose about 6 percent of muscle mass every decade.

Thyroid Hormone

As most of us can attest, an underactive **thyroid gland** isn't always the primary factor contributing to a weight-control problem. The thyroid gland secretes hormones in expending cellular energy.

When people reduce their caloric intake dramatically, metabolically active thyroid hormones decrease, thereby slowing down the body's fat-burning process.

While it is true that the thyroid gland shrinks as we age, even if the standard lab values indicate that your thyroid-hormone levels are within a normal range, you still can't rule it out as a culprit. (Note that I don't recommend that you go out and take charge by introducing supplemental thyroid hormones without professional guidance.) Ideally, thyroid-hormone levels should be near the higher two-thirds of the normal range in order to support weight management.

Thyroid function must be assessed by a healthcare professional, as part of an initial workup when a patient comes in with concerns of fatigue, hair loss, and/or dry skin. Laboratory screening is TSH (thyroid stimulating hormone). The normal range can vary; in the past, the parameters were from 0.5 to 5.0. Currently, endocrinologists (medical specialists who manage hormone-based disorders such as thyroid disorders, diabetes, etc.) recommend that a normal TSH range is from 0.3 to 3.0.

Thyroid function also includes metabolytes derived from TSH, including T3, T4, Free T3, Free T4, and Reverse T3. Armour thyroid is a natural thyroid replacement that can be prescribed by a physician, physician assistant, or naturopathic physician.

A healthy but underperforming thyroid gland can be supported with diet and herbs. Natural sources of iodine to increase energy include Shilajeet Asphaltum puniabinum, Kanchanara Bauhinia variegata, and bladder wrack. Foods that include coconut oil increase metabolism and weight control. Avoid wheat flour, refined sugars, potatoes, and stimulants such as caffeine.

The abuse of thyroid hormone will cause muscle wasting, irregular heartbeat, and profuse sweating. However, a reasonable dosage can be beneficial. If you take a very low thyroid-hormone replacement while on a very low-calorie diet, this will allow the body to convert from carbohydrate-burning to fat-burning, which is not associated with muscle wasting.

Leptin

Leptin is a key hormone, secreted by fat cells, that promotes the burning of body fat and induces satiety. In other words, leptin makes you feel full. The stimulation of leptin from your fat cells curbs appetite and triggers your body to burn calories.

It is sent to the hypothalamus gland in your brain, where it dictates how much fat is stored from your meal. When leptin can't deliver signals to the brain, this is known as *leptin resistance.*

People who have Leptin resistance tend to hold onto their weight, even though they are eating very few calories. If you are overweight, you are likely to be Leptin-resistant. This means that your brain and pancreas don't pick up the signal from leptin that you are full, so when you reduce the amount of calories you ingest, your body thinks you are in starvation mode and slows down the rate at which you burn up food and turn it to energy. So now, leptin's signals aren't getting through. If those messages were reaching the pancreas, it would instruct the pancreas to stop sending out insulin and *start burning fat!*

The good news is that when you increase cardio exercise and build lean-muscle mass through resistance training (such as weight lifting), the cells in your body become more receptive to leptin.

Also, get your sleep! Leptin levels take a nose dive when you don't get adequate restful sleep. When you sleep too few hours, **ghrelin**—a hormone produced in the pancreas—sends out signals for you to raid the refrigerator.

Insulin

Insulin is a hormone that is released from your pancreas when you eat carbohydrates. Insulin's primary function is to control blood-sugar (glucose) levels. When you increase the amount of carbohydrates you consume, you also increase the amount of insulin required. An excess of insulin in the blood could cause a state of insulin resistance, and facilitate the storage of fat. *This is why insulin has been labeled as "the fat-building" hormone.* The remedy? Avoid "bad" sugars or simple carbohydrates such as sucrose, as they cause an insulin spike!

The one essential bit of information that I share with my patients who are seeking to lose weight is that they must build more lean-muscle mass to improve insulin sensitivity, and to help sugar (glucose) transport, in order to reduce the insulin required to maintain a normal blood sugar. *Lower insulin levels will help reduce stored fat.* The body holds onto stored fat when insulin is released, so that it has fat reserved as an energy source.

The first question I ask my patients is, "What do you eat for breakfast?" I bet you can't guess what percentage of patients respond with "Nothing" or "Coffee." I have not kept a running tally, but I can assure you that at least 70% of them state that they just don't have an appetite early in the morning, what with the frantic pace to prepare for work, school or daily activities.

One major influence on appetite control is blood-glucose levels. When you allow a gap of 5 or 6 hours between meals, the blood-sugar (glucose) level declines, triggering the brain's demand for a normal glucose level. This lower level of glucose is behind the desire to consume a sugar source to quickly raise the blood-sugar level. Usually, the quick sugar-fix is a simple carbohydrate or a stimulant (such as caffeine) for instant energy. However, allowing peaks and valleys in blood-sugar levels will eventually have adverse effects on the cardiovascular system.

Resveratrol to the Rescue!

Resveratrol is an antioxidant found in purple grape juice, red grapes, red wine, berries, and cacao. An energy source, it is produced by plants in response to environmental stressors. Plants derive the energy from the sun, soil, and minerals, and are transferred into our blood stream when we ingest them. The best way to absorb this energy source is to ingest it from foods that are high in antioxidant levels.-

Resveratrol improves insulin sensitivity; may improve thyroid function; and powers up your cellular energy house, the mitochondria. This is the component of each cell that produces energy for the body—a function that is enhanced by foods, supplements, or herbs.

Ghrelin

Ghrelin is considered a hunger-inducing hormone. The stomach needs to be full in order to reduce ghrelin levels as well as appetite. Ghrelin is released from Epsilon cells in order to metabolize carbohydrates. The pancreas releases insulin from its Beta cells, in order to metabolize carbohydrates. (The Beta cells and Epsilon cells carry out different functions in the pancreas.) This is how the body controls blood-sugar levels. The body uses sugar for energy. When you consume a huge amount of carbohydrates, they will be converted to sugar. Guess what happens when you consume excessive amount of simple carbohydrates? They are stored as fat in the form of triglycerides—extra fat streaming through your blood vessels!

C ~ Reactive Protein (CRP)

C-reactive protein, or **CRP,** blocks the introduction of **leptin** into the hypothalamus, the area of the brain that controls hunger signals.

The presence of CRP indicates inflammation. Increasing your intake of supplements to foods that reduce inflammation may reduce CRP.

Vitamins and Nutrients That Reduce Inflammation

The following vitamins and nutrients reduce inflammation.

1. Vitamin C
Vitamin C is not internally manufactured by the body, and so must be ingested daily. Because Vitamin C is water soluble, any excessive level of this vitamin in the body is excreted by way of the kidneys. In addition to reducing inflammation, other positive functions of Vitamin C include the growth and repair of tissue that form collagen, and are used to make skin, tendons, ligaments, blood vessels, and scar tissue, just to name a few.

Great sources of Vitamin C include:
Broccoli, bell peppers, kale, cantaloupe, cauliflower, strawberries, raspberries, cranberries, pineapple, lemons, oranges, cabbage, mustard greens, turnip greens, Brussels sprouts, guava, sweet potatoes, and white potatoes, to cite just a few of the most common foods consumed.

2. Vitamin E

Vitamin E is fat-soluble and can accumulate in the fatty tissue (adipose) in our bodies.

Food sources of Vitamin E include:
Almonds, sunflower seeds, sunflower oil, safflower oil, hazel nuts, peanut butter, corn oil, spinach,   broccoli, kiwi fruit, mango, raw tomatoes, turnip greens, dandelion greens, pistachio nuts, and many more.

3. Vitamin D

Vitamin D is a fat-soluble vitamin found in foods. It is manufactured in the body after exposure to ultraviolet rays from the sun. The main function of Vitamin D is to maintain normal blood levels of calcium and phosphorus. Vitamin D aids in the absorption of calcium to form and maintain strong bones. Vitamin D's precursor, calcitriol, promotes normal cell growth, and maintains hormone balance and a healthy immune system. Calcitriol is the biologically active hormone form of Vitamin D. Calcitriol is converted from Vitamin D3 (cholecalciferol) in the liver and kidney. Vitamin D2 (calciferol) is made from ergasterol in plants by the action of sunlight. Vitamin D3 is present in salmon, sardines, mackerel, egg yolks, and liver. A small amount is made in the skin by action of UVB sunlight.

A large percentage of obese patients have low Vitamin-D levels. There is evidence that in obesity, Vitamin D is found in excess in the fatty tissue cells. This might account for lower Vitamin-D levels in blood laboratory screens. In Vitamin-D deficiency, parathyroid levels are elevated. This also corresponds to the elevated levels of calcium in the bloodstream that occur with parathyroid disease.

There is current research to determine whether Vitamin-D deficiency is a result of obesity, or if obesity occurs because of Vitamin D is deficient.

Vitamin D lasts only about 60 days in the body, so you must avoid going for long periods without food or supplemental Vitamin-D intake.

Symptoms associated with Vitamin D deficiency:
The most common symptoms of insufficient levels of Vitamin D may include: muscle pain, weak bones, low energy or fatigue, decreased immune function, insomnia, mood swings, and depression.

Sources of Vitamin D:

There are few natural sources of Vitamin D in the plant kingdom. Many cereals and milk are fortified with Vitamin D. Naturally occurring forms of vitamin D include: eggs, mushrooms, salmon and other fatty fish, fish oils, herring, catfish, steelhead trout, and mackerel.

4. Vitamin K
Vitamin K is a fat-soluble vitamin. Its major role is in blood clotting. Vitamin K is manufactured by bacteria in the large intestines. Deficiency occurs when the body is unable to absorb the vitamin from the intestinal tract, or after long-term treatment with antibiotics. The level of Vitamin K altered with the consumption of dark green vegetables.

(You must consult your physician before supplementing with Vitamin K, if you are on a blood thinner.)

Sources of Vitamin K include:
Spinach, lettuce, kale, cabbage, cereals, some fruits, meats, organ meats, dairy products, and eggs.

5. Niacin (Vitamin B3)
B Vitamins, including **Niacin** (Vitamin B3), help the body cope with stress.

Niacin is water soluble, and therefore requires daily consumption to maintain healthy levels.
Niacin helps regulate metabolism and plays a role in the mechanism to control the level of energy in the body.

Niacin helps enzyme function involved in the production of steroid hormones in the adrenal gland.
It helps the body metabolizes carbohydrates, which are used for energy.

Taking 1,000 mg of Niacin under medical supervision will also lower cholesterol levels. Taking Niacin with other vitamins (such as *Niacin 50mg and Vitamin C 1,000m three times per day*) increases circulation, lowers high blood pressure, lowers total cholesterol as well as the "bad cholesterol," LDL. Niacin reduces triglycerides, thus reducing the incidence of heart attack and stroke. Niacin and niacinamide (Vitamin B3) are found in many foods, such as yeast, meat, fish, milk, eggs, green vegetables, beans, and cereal grain.

Recommended Dosage:
The recommended dose for adults is 10-13 mg daily, and 20 mg in nursing mothers.

What to avoid:
Please avoid excessive niacin intake. It can cause insulin resistance, followed by low blood-sugar. Low blood-sugar (hypoglycemia) will trigger an increase in appetite and lead to weight gain. Niacin can cause so much flushing that it is not practical for most people.

Sources of B3 Vitamins include:
Legumes, meat, fish, peanut butter, and fortified grains. Dairy products contain **Tryptophan,** which helps amino acid conversion into niacin. **Vitamin B6** is needed to facilitate the conversion.

6. Beta Glucans
Beta glucans is a soluble fiber that will reduce inflammation.

Fiber helps increase the feeling of fullness when taken with a meal. It binds to fat and carries the fat out of the body. Beta glucans has been shown in studies to increase **CCK** (cholecystoknin), a hormone that makes us feel full—so, of course, you eat less.

A Good Source of Beta Glucans:
Barley is a good source of beta glucans. It is high in fiber content, and in various minerals (especially chromium), and has a low glycemic index (25).

Testosterone
(And Other Sex Hormones)

Sex-hormone production levels decline with age. This is the most commonly shared factor that influences various body functions. During early development, pre-teens experience physically demonstrable alterations, as sex hormones (estrogen, progesterone, and testosterone) are expressed. Evidence of sex hormones is observed as breast buds in females and, eventually, the onset of menses. Males undergo a change in voice quality (it gets deeper). Both males and females develop hair growth in the axilla (armpits) and in the pubic areas.

Sex hormones are crucial in the maturation of physical development and function. Later, as adults age, they undergo a natural decline in sexual hormone production and their functional activity.

Older men acquire extra fat around the abdomen when *free* **testosterone** levels decline, and excess **estrogen** or *estradiol* levels increase. Some males may convert testosterone to estrogen when testosterone levels are excessive. Therefore, they must be careful to avoid an estradiol level of lower than 20 pg/ml, as this would reduce testosterone's ability to induce fat-cell loss. Weight loss requires the increase in muscle mass in order to increase metabolism to promote weight loss. Inadequate levels of hormones, especially testosterone, interfere with the development of muscle mass. This is why competitive body builders use injections of testosterone and Human Growth Hormone (which is unsafe, harmful, and illegal when not used under medical supervision).

Lower levels of DHEA will also contribute to fat accumulation around the abdomen.

MOVING AND GROOVING TO LOSE WEIGHT

Now that we are equipped with some basic knowledge about how hormones that are produced naturally in our body can influence weight management, we can look at some basic techniques for helping us keep our weight under better control. The main one is *exercise*.

Many people are reluctant to exercise. They feel it's too much work, especially after a long day working, when what's wanted is to eat and rest. And it's true that the gym isn't for everyone. For example, many women complain that gyms are a giant "meet" market. I imagine that's why the concept of "women-only gyms" has gained such popularity.

A Regular Exercise Practice (Ideally) Begins in Childhood

We all are well aware that obesity in children has reached epidemic proportions. With all of the temptation to be current with the latest video game, or to sit at a computer following Facebook, people aren't getting much exercise.

I have had the opportunity to work in Beverly Hills with a pediatrician who designed a weight-loss program for children and their families. It was initially established with a focus on children getting proper nutrition, keeping an eye on portion control, and getting lots of exercise.

Children's school performance is enhanced when their day is broken up with a little exercise. The increased level of physical activity increases circulation—a great mechanism to improve brain function, with the additional oxygen to the brain. The additional *exercise improves mood and reduces anxiety*, due to the "feel-good" neurotransmitter endorphins produced in the brain when the body is engaged in sustained exercise. Additional benefits of endorphin production are that *endorphins reduce carbohydrate cravings.*

At the risk of sounding like my parents, I will say that children aren't as physically active as they were back in the "good old days." While growing up in my home town of Herlong, California, some of us would complain if we missed the one school bus that took us to our schools less than a mile from our home. My parents would repeat the same old story about how, in their day, they had to walk several miles to school back and forth 5 days a week, sometimes in the rain, and they seldom complained. How they picked cotton for 50 cents a day near the plantation where they lived in Louisiana and Arkansas, sometimes with no shoes. My take on that was that they enjoyed that walk to school. It gave them an opportunity to catch up on the latest gossip—and it was not cotton-picking season.

In the 1960s, physical education classes were included in the school curriculum. There were very few, if any, students who failed that class. And it wasn't an easy "A" grade for everyone. Some of us didn't have a natural enthusiasm for sports. Still, we all did our best because it was usually a team effort and you didn't want to let the team down. I recall how, in elementary school, around the start of the school year, we had a national competition in physical education to determine which state had the most physically fit children. We tried to beat the national average in the number of sit-ups and pushups we could complete in 60 seconds. My ranking was average, and that was good enough to save face. Overall, I was clumsy and could not run as swiftly as my class-mates, but I never gave up the attempt to just keep pace.

It wasn't until I was 19 that I finally reached the weight of 100 pounds while taking a "women's conditioning course" in college, and found that I excelled in gymnastics. This gave me more motivation to exercise more. I actually increased my running speed as I achieved better overall conditioning.

It is a travesty that physical education is not a requirement in a balanced school curriculum. I imagine that had I had more exposure to gymnastics in my early childhood, I would have had more enthusiasm about physical education.

Exercising Alone Also Counts

Some of us actually enjoy exercising alone, without any competition, just to use the time for introspective reflection and an opportunity to regroup. I reached my peak in my 40s when I would run with our dog Carmel every morning from 5:30 AM till about 7 AM. We would run (that is, I walked— *she* ran) 1 mile to Staring Lake and then around its 2.3 mile circumference. During the rare exception when temperatures were about 40 degrees below zero Fahrenheit, we'd still manage to run, though just for 20 minutes. I lost some of those extra pounds that I had acquired over the years pretty rapidly. I had not even set out to lose weight. My motive for running with Carmel was to reduce her need to dig under the fence, ruining the neighbor's lawn.

Eventually, walking-running became a little boring. So I mixed it up a bit with attempting to perform chin-ups on a horizontal tree limb that I discovered near the lake on a not-well-traveled path. On the first day, I didn't have the upper-body strength to perform 1 chin up. But after about 3 weeks, I could do *12* chin-ups while simultaneously bringing my knees up. And after 4 weeks, I had dropped 2 dress sizes, although my weight remained unchanged.

This was because I had acquired muscle mass while losing the fat around the gut and butt.

A Panoply of Exercise Possibilities

My patients whom I have advised in weight management turn out to be most successful when they discover an activity that they can enjoy and feel that it is not hard work. Here are some exercise options that are available to you.

Water aerobics is ideal if you are obese. It helps you exercise while reducing the impact on your lower back, knees, and ankles.

A brisk walk daily, starting with a 30 minute walk, as tolerated, works wonders. Gradually increase the distance and the amount of time you walk daily. Most people who don't have physical challenges can accomplish *walking an hour daily.* Many patients claim that they get plenty of exercise because they are walking around at the work place and not sitting a computer for 8 hours per day. When I suggest to them that they must perform a brisk walk and produce some "sweat equity" in order to consider walking as *exercise*, they become annoyed. But exercise, by definition, is *activity that increases your heart rate at least 20 percent (as tolerated), for a prolonged period of at least 20 minutes or more.*

Mowing the lawn with a reel mower is a good cardio workout, if you have a small patch of lawn. and It's great for building up lean-muscle mass. It also helps you to reduce your carbon footprint and your contribution towards global warming.

Gardening: Digging and planting an organic vegetable garden in the spring will not only help you produce Vitamin D from exposure to the sun, but will also provide you with toxic-free food from the Fall harvest.

Dancing—whether by yourself or with a group—is a great way of increasing your metabolism without feeling as though you are working hard. I took a beginner's ballroom dancing lesson, one evening, and had great fun for 4 hours nonstop. I felt it the following day, though. I hadn't danced in years, and could appreciate the enormous *conditioning* you undergo while doing ballroom dancing.

A trampoline, while not for everyone, is a good cardio and aerobic (as well as isotonic) exercise.

Bicycle riding is a sport that the entire family can enjoy. Bicycling can be done by people of all ages . The major advantages of bicycling are improvement in cardiovascular fitness, increased strength, improved balance and agility, increased endurance and stamina, and most importantly *reduced stress*. Don't forget to wear your head gear at all times while riding your bike—remember, safety first. Bicycling at a moderate speed of 12 to 14 miles per hour will burn 235 calories. Gather together friends and family to establish a routine of riding your bicycles 2 hours per day a couple of days per week, and watch those pounds gradually decline.

Spinning is a real endurance booster. You can achieve an overall workout with this activity. Spinning for 45 minutes will allow you to burn 500 calories. Spinning will allow you to build muscle tone. The workout focuses on core muscles, buttock muscles, and thigh muscles. You can work on your abdominal muscles if you maintain the correct position. Spinning can be done year round, is a great stress reducer, and is a low-impact form of exercise.

Jumping rope is part of a workout routine for boxers, who need to acquire fancy footwork in order to move swiftly. A great resource online is Nutri Strategy. (www.nutristrategy.com/activitylist4.htm) They list the number of calories burned while performing various activities. For example, while jumping rope fast for 1 hour, you can burn 708 calories, if you weigh 130 pounds; 844 calories if you weigh 150 pounds; 981 calories if your weight is 180 pounds; and 1117 calories if you weigh 205 pounds.

Nutri Strategy's list also includes some job professions that are naturally high calorie-burning activities. It is a no-brainer that if you engage in activities such as working with a jack hammer, cutting logs, or baling hay for several hours on a daily basis, you might manage to maintain a healthy body mass.

Hula-hooping to music is a workout that you can do alone or with a group. Again, there's no age limit with this activity. I'd advise some caution, though, if you have back problems.

There are so many other fun activities that you can engage in to lose and maintain a healthy weight. Consider these:

- **House cleaning**—especially a nice through cleaning of your floors, down on your hands and knees, where you can see how well you have scrubbed those floor until they are spotless. The results are so rewarding.

- **Cleaning the scum from the bathroom shower glass**— I have a wonderful non-toxic, all-natural solution that leaves the surface squeaky clean (that's in my *nex*t book), and doesn't require a lot of elbow grease.

I have not begun to exhaust the list of possible activities that can prompt folks into moving a little bit more every day and boost their caloric expenditure. So be creative and make up your own list of those activities you would be motivated to perform as part of a weekly routine. None of the activities that I listed need to be done on a daily basis, except some of the housekeeping chores that could be performed just to stay ahead of a long "honey-do list."

Other Weight-Loss Aids

- **Eat well** to have the energy to perform daily tasks.

- Watch your **attitude**, or you might become discouraged and resent the task of exercise. If you frame the task of exercise as a chore, you might not remain as motivated to lose or maintain your weight as you did when you placed it on your "New Year's Resolution " list. I'm not a betting woman, but I presume that most of you can't recall the first 7 items on your list of resolutions. Gymnasiums tend not to be as packed with patrons in the month of March, compared to January.

- **Don't become riddled with guilt** if you don't manage to perform some type of exercise on a daily basis. We're all busy people, with our list of priorities changing daily (if not more often), and thus can inadvertently move exercise to the bottom of the list of daily tasks.

- Another suggestion, if I may: **modify and incorporate some type of isotonic or aerobic exercise while performing some of your activities of daily living,** at home or on the job. One example: if you're washing windows, you could isolate your abdominal muscles and try tightening and then releasing them while deep breathing. Multi-tasking might be a challenge for some of you intense cerebral types, but give it a try. You'd be amazed at the number of activities you can squeeze into your daily routine. For those more economically frugal individuals, you would be amazed at the amount of money you can save by performing household chores yourself. In another book I will share with you some environmentally safe, efficient, and effective cleaning agents you can make from common inexpensive items that you probably already have in your kitchen pantry.

HOW TO EAT AND LOSE WEIGHT

It's not complicated; common sense should be your guide. As you probably know, if you consume more calories than you burn, eventually you will gain weight—that is, unless your basal metabolism is 3500 calories. **Basal metabolism** is the measurement of the amount of energy (calories) used by your body while you are (for example) sitting and reading Facebook. (The Facebook analogy might not be the best that I could choose if you are one of those people who gets very animated while viewing the content on the screen.) In order to lose weight, you must move about with some accelerated, sustained activity for at least 15 minutes daily, and then increase the time by 10 minutes weekly, as tolerated.

Eating a bag of potato chips while sitting at your computer screen is not what I would consider a good practice. You probably would consume more than you were aware of while mesmerized by the computer's activity. So when you are eating, you should concentrate on eating. Relax and relish every bite.

Fundamentals of a Balanced Diet

Let's begin with the fundamentals of what one would consider as a balanced diet, packed full of powerful nutrients. Every meal should consist of a **carbohydrate, a protein, and a fat.**

What are carbohydrates?

Carbohydrates are foods such as breads, pastas, and grains. A balanced diet consists of 30 to 40% carbohydrates. *Complex* carbohydrates are the preferred source; these include fresh fruits, fresh vegetables, whole grain breads, pasta, and cereals.

Carbohydrates are made up of sugars. When carbohydrates are eaten, they are converted to sugar (glucose) in their simplest form, and finally to glycogen and stored in the liver and muscles. Carbohydrates are a primary source of energy for body function.

Complex carbohydrates are slower to convert into its simplest form, when compared to the surge of blood-sugar levels after consumption of a sugar-laden beverage or food. Therefore, I suggest that you avoid simple carbohydrates such as white bread, white rice, and white pasta.

You do want to limit your sugar intake in order to lose weight. I suggest that you limit the list of sweeteners that you use to stevia, honey, or molasses, as they are a better choice than fructose. When patients seek my advice in the weight-loss clinic where I currently work, I ask them to *limit their fruit intake to one serving per day.* I suggest that the shopping list should include items that you generally find in the *outer* parameters of the grocery store (generally where the fresh or non-processed foods are stored).-Very few items on the shopping list would require you to stray very far from this plan and travel down the aisles of a conventional grocery store.

So what items would appear on that list for successful weight management? At the top of the list of healthy carbohydrates are steel-cut oats, whole grain or multi-grain breads, pasta, and cereals, dried beans and peas, brown rice, quinoa, and kasha.

Let's get back to the outer parameters of the grocery store. In terms of produce, the ideal choice would be all organic. However, in these economically challenging times we might overlook the dangers of pesticides and other unhealthy products on mass-produced foods.

When planning for your daily snacks, remember to match carbohydrates with a protein. It is important to understand that when you match a carbohydrate with a protein, the conversion into a simple sugar element is a slower incline and won't be followed by a sudden drop in energy. The best way to reduce urges for quick-energy foods is to keep the blood-sugar levels somewhat even throughout the day.

Now at the risk of repeating myself, need I remind you that excess sugar intake will trigger an increase of insulin release from the pancreas? This is how blood sugar levels are maintained. One of the most practical snack-food combinations to carry while on the go is raw almonds and raisins, or dried cherries.

If you consume too few carbohydrates to perform an activity, the body will start to break down muscle as an energy source. This not a good idea! After all, you do require muscles to move your body about. And the *heart* is a muscle. (You may not have paid attention in elementary school health class when your teacher probably mentioned that.) So be very careful when planning a balanced diet. Just remember, emotional upset isn't the only way your heart can be broken.

Muscle-Building Proteins

Amino acids are the basic building-block of proteins. When we consume proteins, digestive enzymes are released into the digestive tract to break down proteins into amino acids. These amino acids are then structured into muscles, nerves, and organs. Hormones and neurochemicals are also made up of proteins. If your carbohydrate intake is inadequate for your level of activity, the body will break down protein as an energy source.

A case in point is a patient who came to an urgent-care facility where I worked. She was concerned that she might be experiencing a urinary-tract infection (UTI). She stated that she had had a sudden onset of urinary frequency for a few days. She'd had no other symptoms consistent with a urinary tract infection, such as burning, urgent pressure on the bladder, visible blood in the urine, or dark urine color with a strong odor. The nursing staff had obtained a urinalysis and found that all factors of the urine specimen were normal, except for a very high level of protein. Under normal conditions, protein in the urine is not commonly found, except in the case of kidney failure and autoimmune disorders, to name just a few.

I asked her what medications she was taking, and if she had undergone some dramatic change in her diet. Her reply was amazing: she had started a modified Atkins diet just a week prior. She was attempting to lose weight, and because she loved steak she chose to consume steak and eggs for 3 meals a day, and very few servings of vegetables. She reported that she had lost about 7 pounds in a week, and planned to continue this diet for a few additional weeks. I then explained to her that her protein intake had exceeded the capacity of her kidney function, and that protein in the urine is an indication that her protein intake exceeded the levels that her kidneys could filter at that time.

Fats

The recommended daily dietary intake of fat is 20-35 percent of your caloric intake. It's important to realize that *fats* don't make you fat; excessive *carbohydrate intake* is what contributes to obesity, as well as Type 2 diabetes.

"Good Fats" for a Healthy Diet

- **Monounsaturated fats**. These "good fats" are found in canola oil, peanuts, olive oil, avocado, almonds, hazelnuts, pecans, pumpkins seeds, sesame seeds, and cashews.

- **Polyunsaturated fats**. These are found in sunflower seeds, corn, soybeans, flaxseed oils, walnuts, and fish, (salmon, tuna, mackerel, sardines, trout, herring).

- **Omega-3** (a plants source). This is found in chia seeds, walnuts, flaxseed, canola, and soybeans.

"Bad Fats" –Trans fats and Saturated Fats

These are considered to be bad dietary fats, as they contribute to heart disease, and high cholesterol.

Sources of these bad fats are mostly animal sources, which include beef, beef fat, veal, lamb, pork, lard, poultry fat, butter, cream, milk, and cheeses.

The Case Against Eating When You Are Not Hungry

We use food as a central hub of social gatherings. Many people also use food to soothe a broken heart or an injured body part. Celebratory special menus highlight community or family events to recall highlights of the past and hope for the future. Many of us tend to crave carbohydrates when we're feeling sad or "down in the dumps." Emotionally driven preferences for certain foods that help us cope with stressful periods in our life's journey appear to be heavy on the high glycemic-index scale. Perhaps these high-calorie, sugar-laden foods provide us with an instantaneous high, or surge of energy as a "pick-me-up." Many people reward themselves with forbidden foods to highlight mild markers of achievement. A majority of Americans require the ingestion of coffee with cream and sugar to open their eyes and perk up brain function, in order to perform daily work and general activities.

There are many triggers that prompt us to indulge in the consumption of those high-calorie foods. Therefore, the most effective approach in the modification of this behavior is perhaps to choose a carrot instead of a chocolate candy bar. Not an easy task—the knee-jerk reaction is to gravitate towards those high sugar-content foods to provide a quick energy lift.

With the advent of energy drinks, many people select this quick-energy burst instead of healthy foods that provide a steady but slower, more sustained energy. These beverages do not provide nutrients essential in attaining and maintaining good health. Adults must teach by example, if we are to curb the incidence of chronic illnesses that compromise the lives of our children (as well as adults), such as obesity, Type 2 diabetes, heart disease, cancer, and many others. ▪

Let us consider a strenuous workout as a mood enhancer, instead of using carbohydrates as a stress reducer. Endorphins are released into the bloodstream when exercising. Endorphins are mood enhancers that lift our spirits and promote weight control. So when you're feeling down, get a natural high by activating mood-lifting stress-reduction hormones (endorphins) that are released into the bloodstream during strenuous exercise.

OBESE VEGETARIANS

Even If You Don't Eat Meat, Balance Is Needed

There has been a growing trend of many Americans who have converted to diets that omit animal protein. Many of my patients have told me that they object to the treatment of cattle and poultry that are raised on mega -farms in extremely crowded conditions. Some cite not only the adverse impact of the hormones and antibiotics that are administered to the livestock raised in these commercial farming businesses, but also a growing concern about the effects on those humans who consume the flesh of animals that have been raised on genetically modified grain products as feed.

In the weight-loss support center where I counsel people on weight management, some of my patients have attempted to lose weight by omitting animal protein, assuming (like many people) that if they eliminate fat and animal protein from their diet, they will lose weight. While it is true that many vegetables do provide some protein, it is also true that if they are not served with assorted grains, nuts, beans, or legumes, the protein is incomplete and usually results in a deficit of Vitamin B6. While supplementing with vitamins is one alternative, the best strategy is education—the key to avoiding anemia and other adverse health effects. Many patients who haven't adequately researched the *art* of vegetarianism risk some long-term health problems, including obesity and Type 2 diabetes, because they consume too many carbohydrates on the one hand, and not enough protein and healthy fats on the other.

If you want to practice a vegetarian lifestyle, a balanced diet can be achieved. However, it does require some additional planning and preparation, depending on the produce available locally in your community. Factors that must be considered in the decision to go vegan include the *source* of the produce, and how much traveling great distances contributes to the environmental impact of the carbon load. A great economic booster is the growth of local urban farms, as demonstrated in cities such as Detroit.

So many people who hope to lose weight have adopted a low-fat diet . There has been a big commercial push to reduce or eliminate fat from the diet, and most of the general public has accepted this, thinking that it will lead to weight reduction.

But let's get the facts straight: *fats* don't make you fat or overweight! Some fats are actually healthy.

Fats Don't Make You Fat

Healthy fats are needed to optimized brain and hormone function. Healthy fats such as avocado, olive oil, and coconut milk are just a few of the healthy fats that should be incorporated into every meal. Furthermore, you need a balance of fat, protein, and carbohydrate at each meal. When you consume a carbohydrate without a protein or fat, the pancreas releases insulin. Insulin is a hormone that prevents blood-sugar (glucose) levels from becoming too elevated. In digestion, carbohydrates are broken down to their most simple structure (a sugar molecule).This is how the body metabolizes food and converts it to provide fuel for body functioning. The body always attempts to maintain homeostasis—a stable condition. So in this case, it will trigger the *storage* of body fat to be used as a future source of energy. This is the most common cause of obesity in vegetarians who fail to prepare meals that consist of a balance of carbohydrates, proteins, and fats.

What an Ideal Diet Consists of

Typically, an ideal diet should consist of about 35 - 40% proteins, 35% carbohydrates, and 25 - 30% healthy fats. Daily carbohydrate intake for adults should be about 130 grams daily (even as high as 300 grams daily for those participating in athletic levels of activity). The recommended daily requirement of **carbohydrates for** *children ages 1-5* **should be about 290 grams.** Water intake for adult males should be at least 3.7 liters daily, and 2.7 liters daily for adult females. Fats, based on a 2,000- calorie daily intake, should be 20-30 grams (about 30% of caloric intake). Daily protein intake for adult males should be about 56 grams, and for adult females 46 grams.

Sources of Plant-Based Protein

For those who want to want to eat a largely or exclusively vegetarian diet, the following plants rate high in protein.

Amaranth:
Here are some encouraging statistics about what you get from eating 1 cup of amaranth in contrast to other grains.

Amaranth is an ancient grain of the Aztecs of South America. A serving size of ¼ cup contains a laudable 7 grams of protein and is 183 calories per serving.

- 1 cup of amaranth = 129 milligrams (mg) of carbohydrate, while 1 cup of white rice = 148 grams, 1 cup of brown rice = 143 grams, and 1 cup of oats = 103 grams.

- 1 cup of amaranth contains 347 mg of calcium, while 1 cup of white rice has only 52 mg.

- 1 cup of amaranth contains 519 mg of magnesium, while 1 cup of buckwheat = 393 mg, and 1 cup of sorghum = 365 mg, while 1 cup rice contains just 46 mg.

- 1 cup of amaranth contains 15 mg of iron, while 1 cup of white rice has only 1.5 mg.

- 1 cup of amaranth contains 18 grams of fiber, while 1 cup of milled buckwheat = 19 grams, and 1 cup of white rice = only 2.4 grams.

Additional Sources of Plant-Based Protein for Vegetarians

While the following is not a complete list of proteins found in edible plants, it does include the most commonly consumed foods here in America.

In order to obtain a full complement of nutrients and minerals from a plant-based diet, **you need to** understand some basic principles. To avoid anemia, obesity, or Type 2 diabetes, you have to consume a combination of foods needed to achieve a balanced diet. Grains, legumes, nuts, and beans are just a few of the combinations.

Quinoa: 1 cup = 18 grams.

Kidney beans: 1 can = 13.4 grams.

Tofu: ½ cup = 10 grams. -

Soymilk: 1 cup = 7 grams.

Peanut butter: 2 TB = 8 grams.

Seitan meat substitute= 18 - 21 grams per serving.

Black beans: 1 cup = 15 grams. This is also true for pinto, garbanzo, and navy beans. When planning food combinations, remember that 1 cup of cooked pinto beans contains 42.5 grams of carbohydrates; 14 grams of fiber; and a net carbohydrate of 28.5 grams. ("Net carbohydrate" is what is available to be digested, excluding fiber, for example.)

Nuts:
- **Pecans or macadamia nuts: 1** cup = 10 grams.

- **Almonds, whole roasted:** =1 cup 30 grams .

Whole wheat spaghetti: 1 cup = 7.5 grams.

Flaxseed: 1 cup = 31 grams.

Oat bran: 1 cup = 7 grams. -

Essential amino acids (that is, proteins are made up of amino acids) are proteins that are not manufactured in the body and therefore need to be ingested from certain foods. Excellent plant-based proteins are **soy, tofu,** and **tempeh.** Other sources are grains, barley, cornmeal, oats, rice, pasta, whole grains, and bran.

Food combinations that provide a full complement of nutrients are:

- **Grains and legumes**. Legumes are beans, lentils, peas, peanuts and soy products.

- **Black beans and rice.**

- **Pasta and peas.**

- **Multi-grains and peanut butter.**

- **Bean soup and crackers.**

- **Nuts and seeds plus legumes.**

These are the best plant-based food combinations that permit vegetarians to safely avoid animal protein and still remain healthy.

PART II
DIETS FOR SPECIFIC CONDITIONS

RENAL DIET
(To Avoid Kidney Failure)

"Renal" is medical jargon for *kidney*. The most common causes of kidney (renal) failure are high blood pressure and diabetes, if not well controlled. Lupus, an autoimmune disease, is a less common cause. Once people have been diagnosed with kidney failure or near kidney failure, they must limit their intake of foods that are high in phosphorus, sodium, potassium, and purines, because these elements can not be filtered through the kidneys at a rate high enough rate to avoid toxic, fatal levels of accumulation in the blood stream. When the kidneys fail, dialysis is needed to filter out by-products of foods, supplements, herbs, and medications.

Here is a good diet to follow in order to avoid kidney failure:

- **Phosphorus:** daily intake should be no more than 800 - 1,000mg.
- **Dairy:** Milk (unenriched), 8 oz., Brie (1 oz.), sour cream (2 TB), cottage cheese, feta cheese, whipped cream (½ cup), cream cheese (2 TB).
- **Desserts, breads, crackers, grains:** Angel food cake, sherbet or frozen fruit pops, sorbet, lemon cake, sugar cookies, vanilla wafers, pudding (½ cup), white rice, crackers, white bread, cereals, Cream of wheat, Cream of Rice, grits, rice, pasta, bagels, English muffins, couscous.
- **Vegetables:** Green beans, wax beans, potatoes, rutabaga, winter squash, cabbage, beets, cauliflower, carrots, celery, cucumbers, eggplant, peas, lettuce, peppers, onions, summer squash.
- **Meat and poultry:** Beef, pork, lamb, chicken, turkey, fish.
- **Fats:** butter, salad dressing, shortening, vegetable oil.
- **Candy:** Jelly beans, gum drops, hard candy.
- **Beverages:** Lemon-lime soda, ginger ale, cranberry juice, homemade lemonade, homemade iced tea (8 oz.), hot apple cider.
- **Fruits:** Fresh or canned fruit cocktail, canned peaches, plums, and pineapple, berries, and apples grapes
- **Nuts:** Macadamia (12), peanuts (28), walnuts (14 halves).

Foods to Avoid

Corn, parsnips, and sweet potatoes.

Foods Containing Less than 110 mg of Phosphorus per Serving

- **Animal products:** 1 egg, 1 hotdog, 1 fresh sausage, 2 fish sticks.
- **Breads and crackers:** 1 bagel, 1 croissant, 1 English muffin, all crackers (4), 1 tortilla.
- **Cereals:** Cocoa Puffs (1 cup), Corn Chex (1 cup), Rice Chex (1 cup), Corn flakes (1 cup), Corn Pops (1 cup), Cream of Wheat (¾ cup), Kix (1-1/3 cup), Rice Krispies (1-1/4 cup), Special K (1 cup).
- **Carbohydrates:** Pasta (½ cup), noodles (½ cup), rice (½ cups), popcorn (1 cup).

Best Ways to Cook Vegetables to Reduce Phosphorus

Cooking your vegetables leaches out phosphorus. *Steaming or boiling* removes more phosphorus than baking (although boiling does destroy vitamins).

Vegetables Lowest in Phosphorus

Phosphorus intake, for a person in kidney failure or near kidney failure, should not exceed 800mg to 1,000mg daily.

- Asparagus: 56 mg
- Beets: 40 mg
- Broccoli: 66 mg
- Carrots: 44 mg
- Cauliflower: 44 mg
- Celery: 25 mg
- Collard greens: 10 mg
- Dandelion greens: 66 mg
- Endive: 28 mg

- Green beans: {19-38} mg
- Jerusalem artichoke/sunchoke: 78 mg
- Kale: 56 mg
- Parsley: 58 mg
- Parsnips: 71 mg
- Peas: 77- 117 mg
- Pumpkin: 44 mg
- Red cabbage: 42 mg
- Romaine lettuce: 45 mg
- Acorn squash: 14 mg
- Buttered nut squash: 32 mg
- Spaghetti squash: 14 mg
- Tomato: 24 mg
- Watercress: 60 mg
- Zucchini: 32 mg

Foods with Less than 100mg of Sodium per serving

- **Meats:** All meats that are not cured, smoked or processed.
- **Protein foods:** 1 egg, egg beaters, tofu (raw, firm), tuna (low-sodium, 1 can).
- **Breads, cereals, carbohydrates:** Bread (salt-free, 1 slice), Corn Pops, Cream of Wheat (instant or cooked, ¾ cup), Frosted Mini Wheats, pasta, noodles, white rice.
- **Vegetables:** Fresh and canned (without salt), frozen (without sauce).
- **Dairy:** Butter (1 TB), Colby and Jack cheese (1 slice), cream cheese (2 TB), evaporated milk (canned, 1 TB), milk (whole, 2%, 1%, skim), Muenster cheese (1 slice), Neufchatel cheese (1 oz.), Parmesan (grated, 1 TB), Ricotta (1 oz.), sour cream (1 TB), Swiss goat's milk, yogurt, Egg Nog.
- **Desserts, candy, and snacks:** Apple Newtons (2 fat-free cookies), 11 animal crackers (11), ice cream (½ cup), Kit Kat wafer bar (1.5 oz. bar), Mr. Goodbar (1.74 oz.),

Redenbacher Popcorn (2 TB unpopped), rice cake (1), Rice Krispies Treat square (0.8 oz.), Nestles Crunch bar, Nutri Grain bar, Ritz Crackers (5), Snackwell's fat-free Devils Food cookie snack (1), sorbet, Vanilla Wafers (8), Wheat thins (low sodium, 16), Zestidos (11 chips).

- **Condiments and sauces:** Apple butter (1 TB), Bac-Os (1-½ TB), croutons (1 TB), Hellman's mayonnaise (1 TB), honey, horseradish, Mrs. Dash seasoning, mustard.
- **Beverages:** Soy milk, tea.

Reducing Purines

Purines are natural substances found in all body cells, and in nearly all foods. Meats are a source of higher purine content. Uric acid is formed when purines are broken down completely. Elevated uric-acid levels in the blood stream can cause gout attacks, if a person is a gout sufferer. Uric-acid crystals are formed when a person consumes large quantities of high-purine foods, or is dehydrated. Uric-acid crystals can become trapped in the functioning portion of the kidneys and cause kidney damage.

Foods That Are Low in Purines
- **Soups:** Vegetable soups without meat extract or broth.
- **Dairy:** Low-fat cheese, low-fat milk, low-fat yogurt, frozen yogurt.
- **Fruits, juices:** All fruits and juices.
- **Carbohydrates:** Grains, breads, corn cereal, noodles, pasta, waffles, and white rice.
- **Nuts:** Almonds, Hazelnuts, Walnuts, Peanut butter.
- **Miscellaneous:** Gelatin, tea, tapioca, eggs.

Potassium

Foods That Are Low in Potassium
(Less than 150mg per Serving: ½ cup portion, for most servings)

- **Breads, cereals, crackers, carbohydrates:** Breads (any type), bagels, crackers (graham, soda), snack cookies, corn chips, croissants, doughnuts, English muffin, pasta, popcorn, rice, rice cake, hominy, sweet roll, Triscuit, Cap 'N Crunch, Cheerios, Corn Chex, Corn Flakes, Cream of Wheat, Crispix, Grits, Kix, Life, Oat Bran (1/4 cup), Oatmeal, Special K, Wheaties.

- **Vegetables:** Alfalfa sprouts, beans (green, wax), beans sprouts, beets, cabbage (canned), coleslaw, cauliflower, cucumber, eggplant, garlic, lettuce, onion, parsley, peppers, radish, snow peas, turnips, water chestnuts.

- **Fruits:** Apples, apple juice, applesauce, apricots (canned, 4 halves), blackberries, boysenberries, blueberries, cranberries, cranberry juice, Ocean Spray, fruit cocktail, grapes, grape juice, lemons, lime, papaya nectar, passion fruit, peaches (canned), peach nectar, pears (canned), pineapple, plums, raspberries, strawberries.

- **Dairy:** Cheese, eggs, cottage cheese, sour cream.

- **Candy and snacks:** Almond Joy bar, butterscotch, caramel (5 pieces), fig bars, gelatin, ginger snaps, hard candy, Hershey's Chocolate syrup, jam, jelly, Kit Kat bar, Krave Bars, M & Ms (plain), Thank You-brand pudding, Hunt's Pudding Cups, Peanut butter (1 TB), Nestle Crunch bar, Nutri grain bar, onion rings, popsicles, pie (apple, cherry, lemon, pineapple, strawberry, raspberry), sorbet/sherbet, Musketeers bar.

- **Condiments:** Ketchup (1 TB), salad dressing, Mrs. Dash seasoning.

- **Beverages:** Sunny Delight, Tang, Tea 3, Very Fine juices (apple, banana, strawberry).

CHOLESTEROL CHALLENGES AND THEIR TREATMENT

I had the opportunity to work as a primary care provider for the soldiers at the Presidio of Monterey in Monterey, California from 2004 - 2005.

One of the first patients I encountered was a twenty-something, healthy, slender male soldier who suffered from high cholesterol and had been placed on a *statin drug* to reduce his cholesterol level. He had muscle and joint pain, which had become more severe since its insidious onset a few months prior, and he had come in to have an assessment.

Statin drugs include Lipitor, Crestor, and Zocor, which are prescribed to reduce levels of cholesterol. The statin drugs increase liver enzymes, which indicates adverse side effects to the liver function. Since cholesterol is produced in the liver, the statin drugs work directly in the liver to help reduce cholesterol. However, these drugs produce are side effects. Common side effects include painful, stiff, swollen joints of the elbows and knees as well as other joints.

This patient began to experience joint pain about 10 to 14 days after stating the statin drug, and was treated with Vioxx. (Vioxx was removed from the drug formulary after it was implicated in the death of at least 65,000 patients.)

When I asked if the onset of pain could be associated with some type of trauma, he denied having any recent injury or surgical intervention. I then asked if he could recall how long he had been on the statin drug before the joint pain and stiffness became apparent. When I asked him how long he had taken Vioxx for the joint and muscle pain, he looked at me indignantly. He was aware that Vioxx had been recalled after about 60,000 people died of complications related to it. I explained that many of the side effects that he had experienced about 10 days after being started on the statin drugs were clearly listed on the information sheet for Vioxx.

To address his situation, first I had lab tests drawn to assess his total cholesterol levels, as well as a liver-function test to determine his liver-enzyme levels, because the statin drug directly reflected the health of the liver (where cholesterol is manufactured). Statin drugs given to reduce cholesterol levels directly affect liver function. Cholesterol is manufactured in the liver, and statin drugs directly impact the liver. That is why health professionals closely monitor liver profiles for the first few months when starting a patient on these drugs. Until I could fully evaluate the lab results to determine his current liver function, I suggested that the patient stop taking the statin drug and in their place begin taking supplements shown to reduce cholesterol. I also shared with him a list of foods to avoid, as well as the lifestyle changes that aid in attaining the best overall health status.

When the results of his liver-profile report returned, they revealed that his liver enzymes were more than double those in the normal range. And of course, we had opted to stop the drugs weeks before.

A Low-Cholesterol Diet and Treatment

So how did we manage his cholesterol dilemma? Here are the dietary suggestions that I wrote down on a Post-It Note and asked him to follow for a month, assuring him that after at least a 30-day period we would check his cholesterol and liver panel.

- **Oats** daily (oatmeal or Cheerios)
- **Omega-3 fish oil or flaxseed oil** (alternate every few days)
- **Co-Enzyme Q 10.** (This is an antioxidant that helps convert the nutrients from the foods we eat into energy or fuel for basic cellular function.)
- **L-Cartinine.** (This is made in the body from the amino acids *lysine* and *methionine.* **L-Cartinine** is required for the transfer of amino acids into the mitochondria (cellular powerhouse) during the break down of fats, in order to generate energy. **L-Cartinine** boosts energy by stimulating the body's burning of triglycerides as fuel. **L** It allows the body to burn more fat, and to improve stamina and endurance.)
- **Red Yeast Rice.** This is the natural form of Lipitor, and will reduce total cholesterol when taken along with the items listed.
- **Guggulipid.** Guggulipid is an herb that will lower cholesterol levels.
- **Wheatgrass (** 1 ounce daily)
- **No beef** (for the first 30 days)
- **No cow's milk** (can have almond milk)
- **A broad-spectrum Probiotic**
- **30-day colon cleanse**
- **Consume at least one salad daily consisting of 7 colors of vegetables.** Vegetables that are of a darker hue—such as spinach, broccoli, kale, red cabbage, beets, all the darker, richer colors—are higher in antioxidants that scavenge away free radicals (unstable oxygen molecules that can

promote chronic illness and disease). Raw vegetables contain enzymes that are destroyed when the vegetables are cooked. Consuming raw foods is a way of absorbing energy from the sun. The darker the plant pigment, the higher the quality and the more numerous the variety of plants consumed, the more effective the vegetables are in promoting good health.

- **Drink apple-cider vinegar with an equal amount of grape juice (about 3 tablespoons each) 5 minutes before meals.** The energy from eating raw plants is released at its best when enzymes are activated. This bitter beverage tonic stimulates the back of the tongue and activates the body's hydrochloric-acid pump to prompt improved digestion of the meal to follow.
- **Drink lots of water *after* the meal, not during.** Consuming beverages while eating will dilute the digestive enzymes that are necessary to fully release nutrients into the bloodstream. This approach has helped some patients to end the burning acid sensation noticed after consumption of certain foods.

One month later, my patient returned to have lab tests drawn so that we could assess his results since stopping the statin drug and following my recommended diet. He had lost 30 pounds and also had dropped 30 points on his total cholesterol. He reported that the aches and stiffness in his joints had subsided after about 10 days following his stopping the statin drug.

I later learned that several other soldiers at the Presidio, as well as some civilian personnel, had also tried the suggestions that I shared with my patient—and many of them had improved their health profile, including weight loss, lowered cholesterol levels, reduced blood pressure, and much improved sleep.

As I continued to monitor my patient's liver panel, it showed gradual improvement. The numbers were nearly within a normal range about three months after he had stopped the statin drug, and as he continued to consume a diet high in antioxidants to further reduce the inflammation of his liver.

I have shared the above list with many of my patients, family, and friends, and they have reported experiencing better energy, more cognitive clarity, and improved overall brain function.

DIABETES: THE 21ST-CENTURY EPIDEMIC

In this still-young 21st century, we have seen a number of dubious record-breaking statistics regarding the health of American children and adults. For the first time in recorded history, children born in the 1990s are predicted to have a shorter life span than their parents, and to experience an overall decline in their quality of health. The rising cost of health care is due, in part, to the growing numbers of Americans who practice poor lifestyle choices. For example, we don't encourage school-aged children to exercise as part of a balanced lifestyle, as was the case in past generations. We would do better to accept responsibility in developing and maintaining the best possible health practices, permitting us to live out the healthy longevity currently promoted in anti-aging campaigns.

The advent of processed food-stuffs and the increased consumption of these empty-calorie items correlates with the *increase of obesity, Type 2 diabetes,* and *high blood pressure* in children and adults. The phrase, **"Sad American Diet,"** now characterizes the diet that has been exported to developing countries and throughout Europe, where an increase in the percentage of their citizens now suffering from obesity, high blood pressure, heart disease, and diabetes can be observed. Poor dietary choices will result in poor health. Your foods can heal you if you consume a well balanced diet most of the time.

One remedy for these epidemic maladies, which I have heard from physicians who aren't specifically trained in nutrition, suggests that if a certain food taste is appealing, chew it—but then spit it out, because if it appeals to you, it can't be good for your health. Well, there's not much instructional value in this. At the same time, most of the people I treat for eating disorders prefer foods that are processed and contain larger amounts of sugar, salt, and butter—or fried foods that are filled with saturated fats, which contribute to heart disease and predispose people to obesity, diabetes, high blood pressure, heart attacks, and so many more disease processes.

Many of my clients and patients have adopted the notion that they must consume low-fat foods as a weight-control mechanism. One patient realized that by consuming low-fat fast foods in her efforts to manage the weight she had lost, she was retaining fluid. When she discovered that a turkey burger purchased at a fast-food operation was indeed low in fat, yet contained more than 1,000 mg of sodium (salt), she sat up and took notice. As I have repeated to my patients over and over, *fat doesn't make you fat*, when consumed in recommended servings. It's *carbohydrates* in large portions that promote weight gain. This patient understood that the amount of sodium in that one turkey burger was nearly half the total amount recommended in a low-sodium (low-salt) diet. The amount of sodium recommended for people with heart disease— i.e., high blood pressure, heart failure, or kidney failure—should limit their daily sodium (salt) intake to no more than 2300 mg daily (about a teaspoon).

Modest weight loss will reverse signs and symptoms of Type 2 diabetes in most patients. Increasing exercise on a regular basis will also improve insulin performance and reduce the incidence of diabetes.

Foods and Supplements That Help Manage Blood Sugar

- **Alpha Lipoic acid**: Take 600 - 800 mg daily.
- **Stevia** is a natural sweetener.
- **Fish oils** maintain healthy blood circulation and reduce the incidence of retinopathy (hemorrhage of the small blood vessels of the retina of the eye).
- **Camosine:** This is an antioxidant. Take it 3 times per week.
- **Chromium picolinate**: This lowers blood pressure in diabetics. Take 250 - 350 mg daily for females, and 430 mg daily for males.

- **Magnesium:** Foods containing magnesium are green leafy vegetables, meats, grains, and nuts. Magnesium helps support cardiovascular (heart) function. People with diabetes have a higher incidence of heart disease. Magnesium influences the release and activity of insulin. Insulin is a hormone released from the pancreas, and helps control blood- glucose levels.
- **Zinc:** Some foods containing zinc includes lamb, oysters, pecans, almonds, chicken, and sardines. Zinc is necessary for the formation of insulin the beta cells (the functioning cells) of the pancreas.
- **Gamma Linolenic:** Take 270 – 640 mg daily. These herbs have been found to reduce blood-sugar levels,
- **Cinnamon:** Take ½ - 1 teaspoon daily.
- **Salacia oblonga:** This binds to enzymes in your intestines that break down carbohydrates to their simplest form, sugar. Take 1,000 mg daily.
- **Cactus leaves:** Nopales (prickly pear cactus leaves) is commonly found in grocery stores in the Hispanic community. Consumption of Nopales will lower blood-sugar levels in people who suffer with Type 2 diabetes.
- **Benfotiamine:** This liquid form of *thiamine* will reduce neuropathy (nerve pain, usually in the legs and feet). Diabetic neuropathy is a painful condition affecting mostly the legs and feet. The high blood-sugar content in diabetics will cause damage to all body tissues. The damage done to blood vessels in the retina of the eye will break down and leak blood from the small capillaries of the retina. The blood-vessel walls of the legs and feet of diabetics become weak and prone to infection. This is why in the past you would often see diabetics who had undergone amputation of feet or legs because of poor blood-sugar control.
- **Fenugreek:** This herb maintains healthy blood-sugar levels.
- **Ginkgo Biloba:** This herb improves blood flow (take caution if also taking a blood-thinning medication).
- **Astragalus:** This herb reduces incidence of neuropathy (nerve pain).

- **Co-Enzyme Q10:** Take 20 - 60mg daily to improve function of the inner surface of the blood vessels.
- **Psyllium:** Taking 1 tsp. in a glass of water twice daily not only improves blood-sugar levels but also helps lower cholesterol levels.
- **Fruit:** Consume only one serving per day of a fruit (1/2 of an unripe banana = 1 serving). It is suggested that you serve fruit with a protein, such as ¼ cup of yogurt or an egg. Yes, the whole egg—the egg yolk is a good source of Vitamin D. There are more studies ongoing to determine why people with Type 2 diabetes have Vitamin D levels in the lower-than-normal range.
- **Indian herbs:** In Indian food, there are herbs used as seasonings that control blood sugar levels—for example, fenugreek (take 5-30 grams 3 times per day or 90 grams per day).
- **Gurmar Gymnema Sylvestre:** This is another herb, used in India, to help control blood-glucose levels. It reduces blood sugar when 200 – 250 mg are taken twice daily.
- **Pterocarpus Marsupium:** This is a very important herb for the control of blood glucose. The combination of Pterocarpus Marsupium, Gurmar Gymnema, and Tinospora Cordifolia is very important in controlling blood glucose.
- **Chinese remedies:** In China, citizens drink lots of green tea. In addition, some of the herbs commonly used that help with diabetes include: ginseng (1-3 grams), Quei Fu Di Huang Wah, Rou Gui, and Tang Niao Kang. Most of the herbs can be found in herb shops or Chinese medical clinics. All these herbs help regulate blood glucose.
- **Helpful foods:** Some of the foods that also help to control blood sugar include bitter melon, bilberry, aloe vera, salt bush, and garlic.
- **Whey protein:** For people with Type 2 diabetes, this can reduce glucose spikes.
- **Cumin** and **Dandelion** aid in the control of blood sugar.

- **Soluble-dietary fiber:** Consuming this before meals will reduce the amount of carbohydrates absorbed. This fiber can come in the form of psyllium, fruits, and vegetables.
- **Whole grains and complex carbohydrates:** *Avoid* (or *minimize intake of* simple carbohydrates such as white bread, white rice, white potatoes, and white pasta. They incite a sudden rise in blood sugar. Instead, try to eat whole grains or complex carbohydrates. *Always consume carbohydrates with a protein* to reduce sudden blood-sugar spikes. Try to eliminate sugar, fructose, and corn syrup, as these all produce a sudden insulin spike and then a precipitous drop in blood sugar, causing you to experience greater hunger and craving for carbohydrates for instant energy. *Absolutely avoid processed meats,* especially hotdogs! They are loaded with carbohydrates (sugar), salt, and fat, and can increase the risk of diabetes.
- **Increase Vitamin D:** Vitamin D3 can be obtained from egg yolks, salmon, herring, sardines or a Vitamin D3 supplement (about 5,000 IUs—International units—daily). There is also an inverse relationship between Vitamin D3 and weight management. Weight loss of at least 10% will reverse Type 2 diabetes in most cases. When I treat people for obesity, their weight declines when they attain a therapeutic level of Vitamin D3 at 80 mg/dl. Vitamin D deficiency might play a role in the increasing rates of Type 2 diabetes. Vitamin D is associated with reducing the rates of insulin resistance, a major factor in heart disease. Vitamin D is used by the thyroid gland, and secretes a hormone that regulates the body's level of calcium, which in turn regulates blood pressure.
- **Sleep well:** Experiencing regular intervals of good, sound, deep sleep will reduce stress and the excessive release of the stress hormone cortisol. Cortisol is released from the adrenal glands, which are positioned above the kidneys. Cortisol levels peak in the morning for energy, and are at their lowest level at night to help you sleep more deeply.

Cortisol is a sugar that easily converts to fat, which has an affinity to be stored around the gut.

- **Weight loss and management:** Although diabetes would absolutely be reversed by Stem Cell therapy, such a therapy is not currently available as a routine, first-line approach. So let us move forth with some practical techniques that are effective in the management of obesity and that reduce the likelihood of developing diabetes, high blood pressure, and many other diseases related to obesity. (For more on weight management, see the "Weight Management" section of this book.)

- **Lifestyle staples—exercise, diet, and supplements:** You can reverse Type 2 diabetes by means of: daily cardio exercise, along with resistance training to build more lean muscle mass; weight loss, a low-carbohydrate diet; and supplements that support healthy glucose levels.

Part III

MENTAL HEALTH

MENTAL HEALTH
How It Impacts Our Physical Health

How's your mental health, today?

This not a common topic discussed while sitting at the family dinner table. Actually, the topic of mental health is considered a taboo subject. Most of us have not been equipped with the tools necessary to carry on a conversation regarding mental-health concerns that would be of benefit to a family member or close friend. Mental-health disorders and their impact on those close to the suffering person can lead the sufferer to totally withdraw from society.

Depression

Depression is a common problem. It could be situational or short term—usually experienced over the loss of a loved one, for example, or if given a severe medical diagnosis, such as cancer. Most people are able to recover from depression following the death of a loved one in about six months, on average. The announcement of a terminal illness would cause most people to experience stages of emotional adjustments, which might include denial, anger, acceptance, regret, or grief (not necessarily in this sequence).

The ability to cope with depression can vary from individual to individual. Some may find that they are strengthened by spiritual uplift from prayer or meditation. Some find comfort in talking to a therapist, or a friend who is a great listener. Others might benefit from medications designed to reduce anxiety or depression for a short period. Then there are those who attempt to mask the pain or anguish with excessive alcohol intake or illicit drug use.

Bipolar Disorder

Most of us know someone who has been diagnosed with Bipolar disorder. The hallmark of Bipolar illness is extreme mood swings that can vary on a wide scale, going from major depression (including suicidal ideation) to feeling extremely upbeat and impulsive. People with Bipolar illness can become so manic that they are not able to fall asleep for several days consecutively, and may go on shopping sprees, purchasing excessively, or impulsively engaging in high-risk behavior (such as speeding in their vehicle, etc.).

Bipolar disorder is the more recent term for what used to be called Manic Depressive Disorder.
Traditional medical treatment includes prescription medication and psychiatric support.

ADD and ADHD

Attention Deficit Disorder and Attention Deficit Hyperactivity Disorder are disorders that have become very prevalent in the vast number of people, more so in the past 20 years.

There has been more concern in the past decade that teachers might be more inclined to recommend drugs to calm down the activity of a male child whom they consider hyperactive, or for fidgety behavior in the classroom setting. Common symptoms of ADD/ADHD are:

- Trouble starting or finishing a task.
- Difficulty organizing items and schedule.
- Underestimating the time required to complete a task.
- Children with ADD/ADHD exhibit poor self control. They often interrupt others, or blurt out things that have no correlation with subject at hand.
- Adults as well as children with ADD/ADHD have poor impulse control. They are unable to complete a simple task, even if the task requires far less intellect than is true of their knowledge or capability.
- A poor self-concept.
- Being easily distracted.

The toll on the body can vary, when a person with Add or ADHD attempts to cope with or adhere to treatment recommendations. Such a toll may include high blood pressure, chest pain due to anxiety and poor sleep, or depression.

Some Ways to Help with ADD/ADHD:
1. Organize all items commonly used at home and at work.
   - Place items in a designated spot. This greatly reduces the time spent searching for items.

- Label containers "focus," or look at items as you place them so that your ability to recall the location of the item is increased.
- Have a system that provides reminders of meetings, appointments.
- Etc.

2. **Engage helpful allies.** Life coaches or professional organizers and psychologists could be helpful allies in assisting those who suffer with life daily challenges. Getting organized and following through with the task, or the preparation necessary to stay on task, are skills one must work at applying. These activities are not easy adaptations for those who aren't vested in the challenge.

3. **Use promising modalities.** Intervene with modalities not commonly used, such as neurofeedback therapies. The ongoing research regarding the use of equipment that provides an analysis of the brain to identify abnormal brainwaves consistent with a specific malfunction of the brain is a promising treatment modality. This new approach requires a trained technician to operate the equipment. With the use of the computerized analysis, this equipment would deliver the appropriate energy wave to the brain and correct the brain function, reverting it back to normal function.

PART IV

Skin, Teeth, and General Vitality

Acne is an extremely common skin problem during the teen years. It also has been a problem noticed by more adults in their third or fourth decades of life. These ages are transitional stages, marked and influenced by the power of hormones.

Hormonal changes of puberty and declining levels of hormone function as we age affect acne development. Genetics is perhaps the greatest contributing factor. Environmental forces such as pollution, make-up that clogs pores, and sensitivities to foods, cleansers, or lotions that might aid in the propagation of huge carbuncles can also be contributing factors.

I have come across numerous remedies through the years, both as a teen and as an adult who has suffered with various stages of mild to severe acne, that people have claimed helped them to control their acne. These remedies have not always been so helpful!

For example, one 20-year-old female made a very dramatic attempt to clear up a big, red, painful carbuncle on her face, which resulted in a chemical burn. She came into the clinic where I worked, seeking immediate resolution of this problem. When I asked her how it had happened, she told me that she was to be the bride's maid in her best friend's wedding the next day. The day before, she had seen a tiny pimple about to form, and—breaking all the cardinal rules of acne care and how to avoid such a disastrous outcome—she attempted to *squeeze* the little red pimple as it was about to form. Then, as the pimple grew larger and even redder, she *applied abrasive cleansers* in an effort to scrub it away. As the pimple grew even larger, now including nearly her entire nose, in great desperation she took the advice of one of her peers and *applied toothpaste* to the area. The advice was to keep the toothpaste on the skin for *no more than a couple of hours.* So she assumed that if two hours should do the trick, then perhaps overnight would be even more effective. Yes, she intentionally kept the toothpaste on the pimple overnight—only to discover the next morning, with much horror, that she had managed to burn and remove the skin covering this very large carbuncle, which was now redder, more painful, and positioned right in the middle of her face. Clearly at this juncture there were very few remedies that would resolve this dilemma overnight.

I instructed her to avoid any abrasive scrubs for the next week and not to disrupt the scab that would soon form to protect the area from bacterial overgrowth. I gave her a prescription for antibiotics, and suggested that she use a mild, nonabrasive wash, followed by a toner and an oil-free moisturizer. She could apply a mineral-powder foundation containing zinc to heal the skin, which also would function as a natural sunblock. For future acne care, I gave her a list of the best tricks used with relative success to minimize and manage breakouts. Many of these tactics, I acquired as an acne sufferer, myself, though most came from my training as an esthetician. I presumed, rightly, that the information I gained while training to become a licensed esthetician would enhance any care I could provide to my patients regarding an array of dermatological issues.

I have applied much of what I learned as an esthetician to my patients' education, and have helped those with acne reduce the frequency and intensity of acne flare-ups. As a Physician Assistant, my primary goal is to provide effective acne treatments while avoiding medications such as Accutane. As a healthcare provider, I have sought to uncover the *root cause* of a disorder and to eradicate the underlying factors that contribute to the problem. My additional training as an herbalist has also played a role in the successful outcomes for a variety of disorders.

Remedies to Treat or Prevent Acne

Water: Water, water—drink lots of fresh, clean, sugar-free water. You should consume at least eight 8-oz. glasses per day. The skin is the largest organ of the body. When you eat and drink food and liquids to provide fuel for the body, when the body has finished processing and using this fuel, byproducts called *waste products* are produced and must be excreted from the body. The *liver* is responsible for the process of breaking down food into a form that the body can use. This process is called *metabolism*. The *kidney* excretes byproducts in a liquid form called urine. If you consume only a small amount of liquids, the kidneys release smaller volumes of urine, causing more stress on the kidneys. Constipation occurs due to very dry stools collecting in the intestines. The higher concentration of urine (due to not drinking sufficient water) and the slower-moving stool will cause higher levels of toxic byproducts to build up in the bloodstream, eventually causing problems with all the organs and their ability to function well. Ultimately, the skin will suffer because these waste byproducts must be released from the body somehow. The result is acne, general body itch or rash, and dull, unhealthy appearing skin.

Exercise: This is crucial for everybody. Producing sweat is a great way to release an accelerated amount of toxins from the body. That's why your skin appears to glow after a vigorous workout and shower. Endorphins are released in the bloodstream when you exercise, which helps in stress reduction.

Rest: Improved rest can assist not only with better sleep but also a better-functioning body and better-looking skin.

Eating clean foods: Raw foods are the best. When you cook foods, you destroy the enzymes that are naturally present in raw fruits and vegetables. Enzymes are important for the digestive process in breaking down the foods into their simplest form, therefore causing less stress on the liver's metabolism. Digestive enzymes are released in small amounts from the pancreas, the liver, and the gallbladder. Smaller amounts of digestive enzymes are produced and released as we age (that's why as we grow older we are less able to tolerate foods that we ate when we were younger). I instruct my patients who are seeking to lose weight, both children and adults, to consume mostly raw foods so that the body burns cleaner fuel. Ideally a total of 7 colors should be represented in the salads and fruits they consume daily. (See the recommendations in

"Cholesterol Challenges and Their Treatment.") The darker the colors of fruit and vegetables contain higher levels of antioxidants. Antioxidants play an important role in scavenging away the metabolic byproducts produced in the digestive process. The best foods to consume for great skin are those that support overall body function. Healthy looking skin is usually reflected in the quality of the skin's appearance. Most patients ask for a list of foods. Since I am not a registered dietitian, I offer up a broad list:

- Greens
- Grains
- Seeds
- Fish
- Red meat (in limited amounts)
- No cow's milk (you can have almond milk).
- Avoid sugar at all costs (although following this last suggestion to the letter is nearly impossible, as most processed foods contain sugar in some form)

Supplements: These include Biotin (2,500 mcg daily); zinc (5 mg); magnesium (100 mg); calcium (400mg); and potassium (at least 4.7 grams). These are the most crucial, and can be found in a whole-food diet. Magnesium, calcium, potassium, and other nutrients can be found in tomatoes. Greens such as Spirulina, barley, broccoli, cabbage, kale, parsley, kamut, wheat germ, alfalfa leaf, and dandelion root contain all the minerals needed to support skin health as well as overall general good health ,because they support all the organs of the body.

Good fats: Avocado, nuts, and olive oil support both skin health, and brain and hormone function.

Protein: Beans, peas, and lentils are good sources of protein. However, remember that some beans are also high in carbohydrates, so be sure to watch those carbohydrates if you are diabetic or if you are attempting to lose weight.

Hormones: Hormones play a big role in the development of acne, if you are genetically predisposed to acne. Some women enjoy the benefits of fewer acne outbreaks while taking certain birth-control pills. The changes that occur during the teen and the perimenopausal years are influenced by hormonal changes.

Basic skin cleansing for acne-prone skin can be a challenge, depending on the stage when a pimple might likely surface. One of the most effective approaches includes the use of a glycolic cleanser. Glycolic cleansers are made with vitamin A extracted from fruits. The reason why glycolic cleaners are so effective is that they promote a more accelerated turnover of the outer dermis of the skin. The faster the skin turns over (or exfoliates), the less likely the pores will become clogged. The reason acne-prone skin is susceptible to the development of pimples is not because of one single factor. The sebum (oil) {is more profuse, and tends to be of a thicker composition and more likely to clog the pores. Now you have a clogged pore, which will shed the outer dermal skin, and environmental dirt will collect within the pore. Soon, bacteria will begin to grow and a pimple will then develop. As the body attempts to reduce the spread of the bacteria into the deeper tissues, it will form a capsule around the pore to encase the bacteria. The area becomes red, warm, and enlarged as bacteria grow, and the body dilates blood vessels in the area to send more blood, carrying oxygen nutrients and white blood cells to fight the invading bacteria. The pores of the skin become larger, and increase the development of blackheads. These develop when excessive oil, shed dermal layers of skin, and dirt collect. When the sebum is exposed to air, the oil oxidizes and turns black.

Keep your hands away from your face. Remove makeup before you fall asleep for the night. Only use moisturizers without oils that clog pores.

The Best Skin-care Routine to Control Acne

- 7% glycolic wash or cleanser, twice daily.
- Use a toner to provide an acid mantle and reduce bacteria growth.
- Oil-free moisturizer.
- Bentonite clay mask, twice weekly, to better control oil production.
- Facial (monthly): steam, followed by a medicated mask; galvanic current to lift blackheads.
- Drink lots of clean water.
- 7 servings daily of vegetables and 1 or 2 servings of fruits.
- Change your pillow case every other night to avoid exposing your face to an oily, bacteria-filled pillowcase.
- Exercise to sweat and remove toxins.
- Infra-red sauna (monthly) to detoxify your body. Removing heavy metals is also *anti-aging.*
- Remove all make-up at the end of the day.
- Don't squeeze pimples.
- Take biotin (at least 2,500 mcg daily) to support healthy skin, hair, and nails.
- After you have used a glycolic wash for 6 weeks, find an esthetician that can apply a "Jessner Peel." Dr. Jessner's peel contains several different acids, including a glycolic acid.

HEALTHY TEETH FOR A HEALTHY BODY

Unhealthy Teeth Can Cause Other Problems, Too

Gum disease (*periodontitis*) is associated with heart disease. Bacteria in the mouth can spread to the bloodstream. Gum disease is linked to heart disease by inflammation. Inflammation is the collection of signs of an infection, including: red, hot tenderness; swelling. This is called *chemotaxis*. When the body detects an invasion of a foreign body or infection, it will respond by dilating the blood vessels. This increases the inflow of the white blood cells so they can fight off an infection and wall off the invader to prevent spread of the infection or deeper invasion of the foreign body.

Chemicals that promote inflammation contribute to *atherosclerosis*, an inflammatory disease that affects the inner lining of the arteries. In this condition, the inner lining (endothelium) of the arteries becomes thick and stiff. Inflammatory gum disease also is linked to cardiovascular episodes of strokes.

Obesity is a risk factor in periodontitis, gingivitis, dental caries, and conditions associated with Metabolic Syndrome (Syndrome X), which includes high cholesterol or triglycerides, insulin resistance, high blood pressure, and Type 2 diabetes. All these can worsen periodontitis.

There is also a significant relationship between periodonitis and osteoporosis.

In pregnancy, oral infection can increase the risk of low birth-weight in newborns. Pregnancy can increase the severity of gingivitis.

It is best to have a tooth removed, once it has decayed.

How to Maintain a Healthy Mouth

Good oral hygiene is essential for long-term good health. Brushing your teeth after every meal and snack is an excellent practice, although it's not always followed (perhaps due to the inconvenience of carrying a toothbrush and toothpaste with you).

It is also important to do regular dental flossing, brushing the tongue and inner cheeks (buccal mucosa), deep cleaning, and regular dental checkups. These preventive approaches are essential for-maintaining healthy teeth and gums.

Several practical remedies and techniques can reduce inflammation and strengthen gums:

- **Co-Enzyme Q10:** When applied directly to the gums of the teeth, it will reduce gingivitis, reduce the occurrence of bleeding gums, as well as reduce the gum-pocket depth.
- **Essential oils:** Oils such as Tea Tree oil and eucalyptus can kill bacteria and fungus.
- **Clove oil:** Cove oil reduces pain and inflammation.
- **Green Tea** has an antioxidant called *catechins*, which can reduce the incidence of plaque and bacteria.
- **Aloe Vera** is a remedy that reduces ulcers in the mouth.
- **Vitamin C** can aid in the prevention of gum disease and tooth loss.
- **Vitamin D plus calcium** (800mg daily) can reduce the risk of periodontitis.
- **Omega 3** (about 3,000mg daily) and **Omega 6 from Borage** (3,000mg daily) can reduce inflammation and gingivitis.

Heavy Metals in the Mouth

An additional concern is dental cavities filled with mercury or other heavy metals. When the metals content in dental fillings are disrupted by way of extraction, these metals leach into the blood stream and are deposited into organs, including the brain.

Chelation with EDTA will remove most heavy metals from the blood stream. We administer Glutathione 2000 mg intravenously 3 or 4 times per week for 3 months, and then weekly for one month. Glutathione is an antioxidant. It breaks up heavy metals, which are usually stored in fat cells, then excreted out in urine and feces.

AN INFORMED PATIENT IS A COMPLIANT PATIENT
Understand Your Medications, Take a Holistic Approach, and Practice Preventive Health Care

Patient education is pivotal in the management of chronic illness. Patients who are diagnosed with a chronic illness must be given information that they can make use of to reduce complications related to disease progression. In conventional Western medicine, many disorders are traditionally managed with chemical medications, which all have potential side effects. Unfortunately, patients who are not compliant with medications and who have not been educated in proper dietary practices could suffer with complications from taking these medications—complications that may progress to include severe illness.

When I worked as a nurse in an Intensive Care unit, I recall caring for a male patient who was only in his mid-30s who had suffered several strokes and major heart attacks. This had happened because he failed to take his medication for hypertension. One of his objections to taking the medication was its side effects, including an inability to achieve an erection. Additionally, he had very little information-about appropriate nutrition, or that his stressful career might have affected his health adversely. The patient's mother told me she had pleaded with her son to comply with the medication prescribed, as well as to lose some weight, engage in regular exercise, and reduce his salt intake. Years before, after surviving a minor heart attack and receiving many prayers from fellow church members who visited daily and prayed with him, laid healing hands on him, and sang hymns, he had not suffered severe problems. Certainly, the spiritual component was uplifting and had played a role in his recovery; but his failure to fully comply with *all* aspects of lifestyle changes needed to maintain a normal blood pressure were catching up with him. Had he been willing to learn about the components of a healthy lifestyle and follow the best guidance of the day, he likely could have easily avoided the complications he suffered from, and at such a young age.

Patients who are informed will usually make better choices about their health and lifestyle options. All patients should be given adequate information regarding disease management so that they can fully participate in making the best decisions possible.

A Holistic Approach to Disease Prevention

Patients and their families should be encouraged to adhere to as many relevant aspects of health management as possible, including information about disease *prevention*. A holistic approach to disease prevention should include all elements that would support the whole person—that is, all components of the physical body, spiritual support, and emotional stability should be addressed as a whole. When people are upset emotionally, it can affect their heart rate or blood pressure.

I always ask my weight-management patients about their quality of sleep in general. I explain that chronic sleep deprivation can raise their levels of cortisol (a "stress" hormone released from the adrenal glands). Cortisol sends sugar to the muscles in times of stress, charging us with super energy to fight or to run very fast to flee from danger (the "fight-or-flight" syndrome). Cortisol was very useful when cavemen had to chase down their food and drag it back home. However, since we are not engaging daily in such marathons any longer, when we experience this super-charged level of stress, it stays in our system and can wreak havoc with our health. (For more details on cortisol, see the chapter on "Weight Management and Hormones.")

Prevention is the best approach in caring for our health. Consuming the proper diet, making sure to get regular exercise, avoiding toxic pesticides, drinking clean water, and avoiding smoking and excessive alcohol intake all are important in healthcare maintenance. Our emotional well being, as well as spiritual integrity, is integral to reducing disease.

FULVIC ACID
A Miracle Molecule

Many of us are well aware that our vegetables and fruits have been depleted of life-promoting nutrients because of the use of commercial fertilizers. Studies have indicated that our vegetables and fruits are depleted of minerals and vitamins because the soil has been depleted of minerals. The use of commercial fertilizer has killed off the organisms necessary to convert soil into humus containing life- promoting nutrients. Mass production of foods has left many of us seeking out a variety of vitamins and supplements to replace the elements missing from crops grown in highly fertilized soil.

In the remote past, foods could truly heal; but this is no longer the case in many parts of this country. We now have foods that have been genetically manipulated, depleting the original quality (or quantity) of minerals and vitamins contained in foods that are grown naturally. This is a case where increasing the volume of foods produced in an artificial environment might *not* result in life-giving foods.

Fulvic acid is a vital mineral—found in organic plants and soils—that I refer to as a "miracle molecule." A single molecule of fulvic acid can carry 60 or more minerals and trace elements into the cells.

Here are just some of the other "miraculous" properties of fulvic acid:

- **Fulvic acid can balance and energize cell life** by increasing the energy in each cell. Enzymatic action is the life force behind vitamins and nutrients. The action of enzymes is necessary for metabolism. Fulvic acid extends the amount of time during which nutrients remain active by increasing the availability of essential nutrients. It is an antioxidant and a natural electrolyte, and it helps rebuild the immune system by increasing the bioavailability of nutrients and minerals.

- **Fulvic acid is an effective treatment for wounds, burns, and rashes**, and can neutralize poison ivy and poison oak.

- **Fulvic acid can neutralize radioactive and toxic waste, scavenges heavy metals,and detoxify pollutants.** Many people who live near nuclear-material sites or downwind from nuclear sites would benefit from fulvic -acid intake. Fulvic acid has been used in Europe for decades, only recently receiving FDA approval here in the United States.

Fulvic acid is found in humus and can be found processed into a liquid tincture. A few drops are placed into a few ounces of water.